Wild
WORKOUT
BEAUTYFLEX WORKBOOK
Bring out the Animal in You

The **FORYSTEKS'**

Wild WORKOUT BEAUTYFLEX WORKBOOK

ISBN: 978-1-935986-21-8

Published By:

LIBERTY
UNIVERSITY.
Press

1971 University Blvd.
Lynchburg, VA 24502
www.liberty.edu/libertyuniversitypress

www.MyWildWorkout.com

TABLE OF CONTENTS

How to use this Journal .... 4 - 5

Sample Journal Pages .... 6 - 7

Four Secrets of Health .... 8 - 11

Before and After Photo Page .... 12 - 13

WildWorkout BeautyFlex Journal planning pages .... 14 - 125

HOW TO USE THIS JOURNAL

The purpose of this journal is to get you on track to a healthy lifestyle by increasing your awareness of the choices you are making regarding your daily exercise as well as what you are putting into your body. You will be amazed at what you are actually putting into your mouth as well as how often you are putting something into your body. Keeping a journal brings to light exactly what's going on with your body.

The drinks and foods you consume are the materials your body uses to rebuild itself on a daily basis. When you give your body the best materials to do its job, you will find healthiness. Your body will begin to look and feel fantastic! Filling your body with subpar building materials to work with is similar to a crooked homebuilder who uses scrap lumber and

Styrofoam blocks instead of quality lumber and concrete blocks—the house will not be what it should be.

Making healthy choices when exercising, drinking, and eating is easy, and as you log your building materials in this journal, you will begin to see where you can improve the quality of the materials you are giving your body to work with.

You'll also begin to recognize harmful materials you have been sneaking into your body that are actually breaking it down, destroying what you have been trying to build. Identifying these will allow you to replace them with better choices that will work with you and help you build the body you want.

Your goal is to drink eight glasses of pure water a day—reducing and working towards eliminating your sodas and sugary drinks. Your goal is to have your food prepared in ways other than frying or deep fried.

Your goal is to replace white bread, white sugar, and white flour, with the much healthier choices taught in the *Four Secrets of Health*, while partaking heartily in healthy choices and many healthy snacks!

We're not a fanatic on all of these things and realize we all have to live in the real world. I believe in the 80/20 rule—if you follow the rules 80 percent of the time, you can slide 20 percent of the time and still be all right. I know there will be times when you'll eat an unhealthy pizza that would knock over a rhinoceros. Just make sure you are following the 80/20 rule, and make sure you don't slide into it becoming 20/80!

Also, don't be afraid to order a salad once in a while. The closest some people ever get to a salad is when they cut the grass. Get a salad with vinaigrette or a light dressing, and you'll love it!

Refer constantly to the *Four Secrets of Health*. They are so simple and so effective.

Use your Wild Workout exercise course for your daily exercise routine. Write down in the journal what exercises you did, what approach was used, what you drank, what you ate and how it was prepared, and what you snacked on. At the end of day, truthfully fill in the yes or no boxes. Strive for all boxes to be truthfully marked yes, and give yourself a grade for the day so you can always have a reference to see the progress you have made! My friend, you will then discover how awesome your body can be, and you'll be amazed at how quickly it responds!

Week 1 Day 1
Date: 11 /04/ 25

Wild WORKOUT.

Approach Used

☐ Direct Target ☒ Mix & Match ☐ Circuit

Wild WORKOUT. **Exercise**

Exercise	Reps	Sets
Panther Flex I	15	3
Dolphin Flex I	15	2
Frog Flex II	20	1
Eagle Flex	20	2
Bear Flex I	15	2
Shark Flex II	25	2
Horse Flex III	10	3
Kangaroo Flex I	10	2
Elk Climb	12	1
Cheetah Dash	8	1

Self Evaluation: (Check one) ☐ A+ ☒ A ☐ B ☐ C ☐ D ☐ F

Tommorrow strive for A+

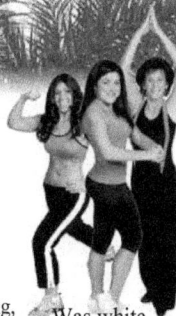

Hydration
12 oz Glasses of Water

☒ ☒ ☒ ☒

☒ ☒ ☒ ☒

Food	How was it Prepared?	What Dressing, Topping, dipping sauce, or butter was used?	Was white flour or sugar used?
Whole Wheat Bagel	Toasted	Butter	No
Turkey Sandwhich	Grilled	Mustard	No
Broccoli	Steamed	Cheese	No
Salmon	Baked	Lemon Butter	No
Mashed Potatoes	Boiled	Brown Gravy	No
Baby Carrots	Steamed	None	No
Side Salad		Vinaigrette	No

	Yes	No
Did I follow the "Four Secrets of Health" today?.....	☒	☐
Did I keep myself hydrated today?..........................	☒	☐
Am I Proud of my workout for the day?.................	☒	☐
Did I snack Healthy today?.....................................	☒	☐

Snacks and Beverages:	Candy, Sugar, or Salt Coated	Dipping Sauce	Healthy or Unhealthy
Black Coffee	No	None	Healthy
Sliced Apple	No	Peanut Butter	Healthy
Chocolate Peanuts	Yes	None	Unhealthy
Raw Almonds	No	None	Healthy
Fruit Smoothie	No	None	Healthy
Banana	No	None	Healthy

4 SECRETS OF HEALTH

There are four secrets to health that are *so simple, yet so effective*—constantly refer to them, practice them, and make them part of your lifestyle, and you will be amazed at how easy it is to be and remain healthy! Being healthy is not found in trying out fad diets and chasing fancy and expensive trends. It is making solid healthy decisions on a consistent basis. Being healthy is a lifestyle, and when these four secrets become a part of your regular decisions, they will make all the difference in the world. Take them seriously and make them a part of your life starting today.

SECRET #1—EXERCISE

The human body was created to last a long time. It's one of the only things in the universe that gets BETTER the more you use it! Experts agree that exercise will help:

- Keep your weight under control
- Reduce your risk of heart disease, diabetes, and high blood pressure
- Improve your blood cholesterol levels
- Prevent bone loss
- Boost your energy levels
- Manage tension
- Improve self-image
- Control anxiety
- Control depression

Exercise on a regular basis. The only things that don't move are rocks and the dead! Exercise regularly. You now have BeautyFlex®, which can be done anywhere at anytime, so NO EXCUSES!

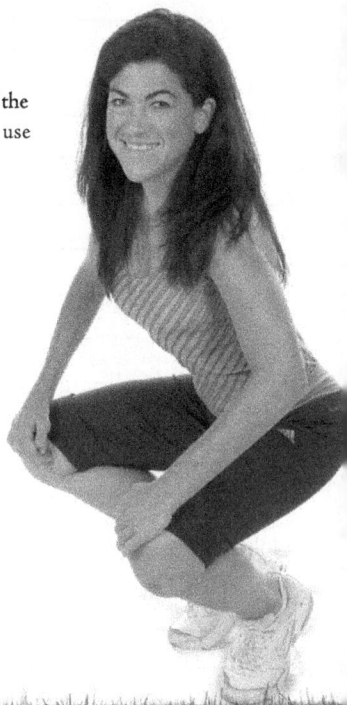

SECRET #2—DRINK ENOUGH PURE WATER EVERY DAY

Experts agree that our bodies require a minimum of at least eight glasses of pure water a day. If you are very active and involved in strenuous exercise, you should drink much more than that. After all, seventy percent of your body is made up of water—not protein, not carbs, not meat, or anything else. PURE WATER is liquid life. Through daily sweating, breathing, carrying oxygen to muscles, helping to digest food, flushing waste products from the body, lubricating joints, and *so* much more, *so* much of our water is lost daily. Even if you are a couch potato, your water level must be replenished—eight glasses a day minimum.

The next time you are at the store, and your hand is reaching for a soda, say, "No. I will grab a water drink instead." It is now available everywhere in a variety of forms—spring, artesian, natural, bottled at source, carbonated, flavored with pure fruit juices, in a bottle, in a can, by the gallon, six pack, case—at the office, delivered to your home in five-gallon jugs. It's everywhere. So there is no excuse to not pass on the soda and sugar drinks and drink eight glasses of pure water a day. It's more important than your diet. Because seventy percent of you is water, give yourself a break and drink some!

SECRET #3—STAY AWAY FROM WHITE BREAD, WHITE SUGAR, AND WHITE FLOUR

Experts agree that there are many healthier choices than "white" foods:

White bread—rather, choose whole wheat, whole grain, rye, pumpernickel, multigrain, etc.

White sugar—rather, choose honey, brown sugar, unprocessed cane sugar, etc.

White flour—rather, choose whole wheat noodles, spinach noodles, brown rice, etc.

It's the processing, bleaching, etc. of the white products that make them an unwise choice. Many people have pounds and pounds of waste stuck in their intestines because of their poor diet of these types of foods—plus they are clogged!

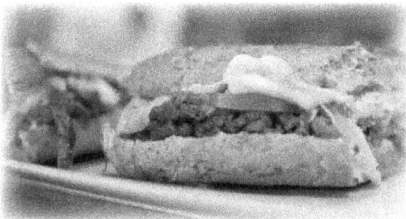

The healthy choices are not only good for you and add nutrients to your body, but they also help to keep you clean inside and properly cleansed within. The healthy choices are everywhere and conveniently available from supermarkets to restaurants. So no excuses—choose healthy.

Ask for a whole wheat bun for your burger. Yes, the fast food places will give you one. You only have to ask. Ask for whole wheat noodles with your pasta. Ask for spinach noodles, ask for honey, ask for a whole wheat crust in your pizza. Get your sandwich on multigrain bread. You have not because you ask not! No excuses!

SECRET #4—EAT BAKED, NOT FRIED

Experts agree that the frying of foods is what soaks everything full of grease, fat, and lard! Go for a baked potato, not French fries. Go for baked chips, not fried. Go for baked, grilled, broiled, or flame-broiled lean meat, fish, turkey, steak, or chicken—anything but fried and deep fried.

Use virgin olive oil instead of lard. It's your choice. Make it—no excuses! Plus you can snack all you want, if you snack on the right healthy foods.

Here's a list to help you:

FRUITS

Apples	Oranges
Plums	Kiwi
Coconut	Nectarines
Tangerines	Berries
Strawberries	Raspberries
Melons	Grapefruit
Grapes	Bananas

VEGETABLES

Cauliflower	Broccoli
Carrots	Green peppers

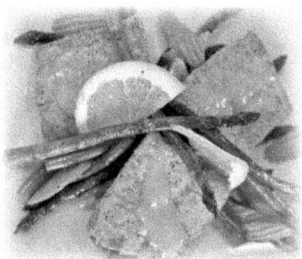

Lettuce	Cucumbers
Peas	Beets
Celery	Cabbage
Green beans	Radishes

RAW NUTS and SEEDS

Sunflower seeds	Almonds
Cashews	Walnuts
Hazel nuts	Brazilian nuts
Hickory nuts	Peanuts in the shell

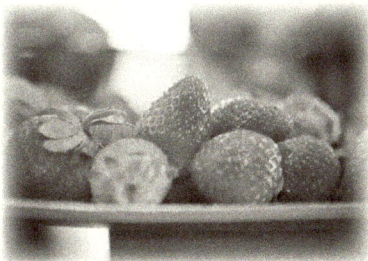

Just be careful you are not loading up your snack choices with fattening sauces and dips and that the seeds and nuts are not coated with salt or candied. Every grocery store now has a wide selection of these healthy snacks, so go load up on them. Leave your excuses behind!

Name:_____

Weight:_____

Height:_____

Age:_____

Waist:_____

Chest Size:_____

Hip Size:_____

Other:_____

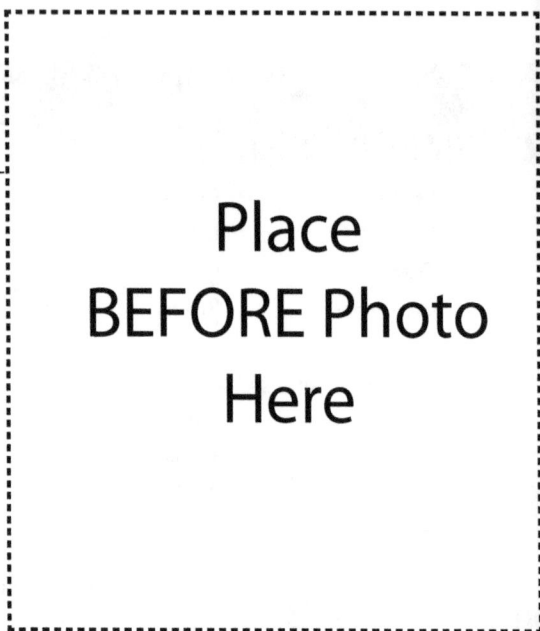

Date:____/____/_____

Name:_____

Weight:_____

Height:_____

Age:_____

Waist:_____

Chest Size:_____

Hip Size:_____

Other:_____

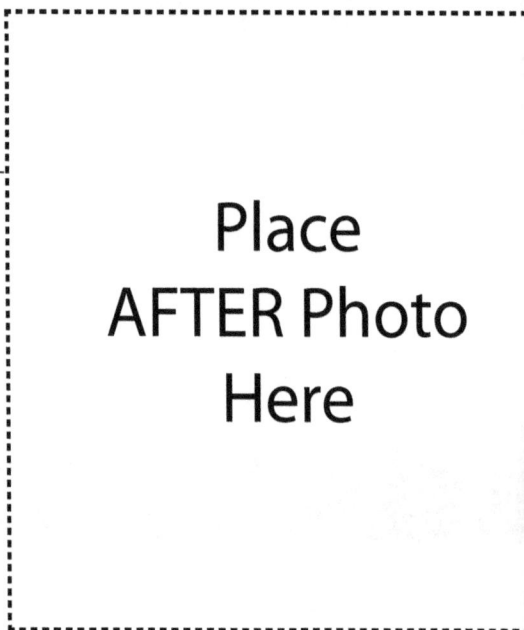

Date:____/____/____

For ALL your exercises and routines
Refer toWild Workout BeautyFlex

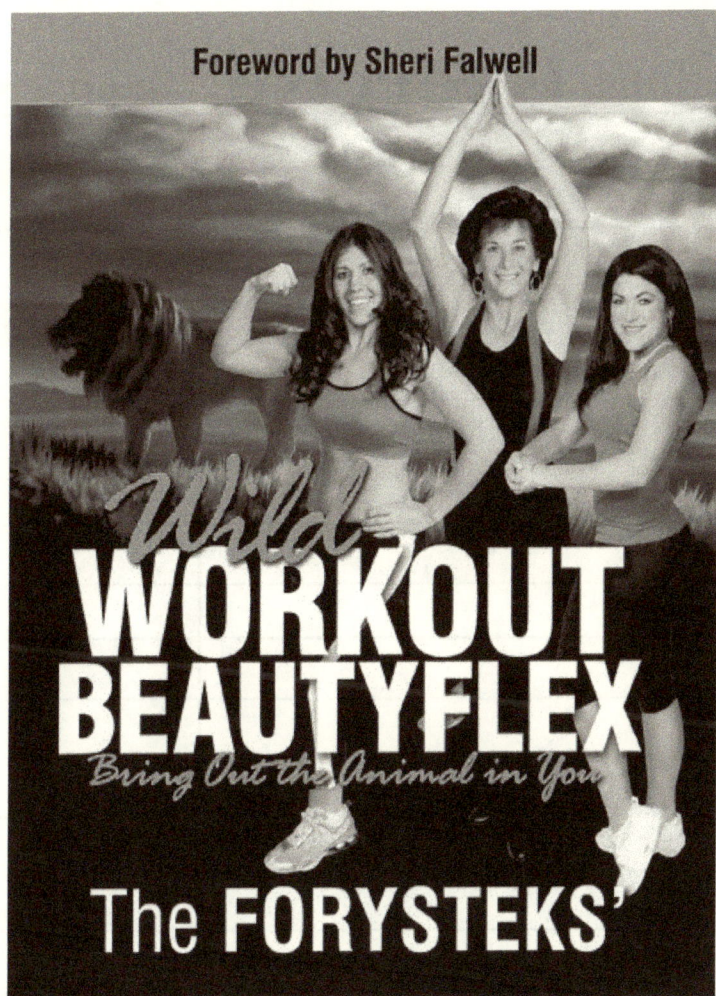

Foreword by Sheri Falwell

Wild
WORKOUT
BEAUTYFLEX
Bring Out the Animal in You

The **FORYSTEKS'**

Visit www.MyWildWorkout.com
And talk with the authors
with all your questions
and comments about Fitness

Wild **WORKOUT**®

Approach Used

☐ Direct Target   ☐ Mix & Match   ☐ Circuit

Wild **WORKOUT**® **Exercise**

Exercise	Reps	Sets

Self Evaluation: (Check one) ☐ A+ ☐ A ☐ B ☐ C ☐ D ☐ F

Hydration
12 oz Glasses of Water

☐ ☐ ☐ ☐

☐ ☐ ☐ ☐

Food	How was it Prepared?	What Dressing, Topping, dipping sauce, or butter was used?	Was white flour or sugar used?

	Yes	No
Did I follow the "Four Secrets of Health" today?.....	☐	☐
Did I keep myself hydrated today?............................	☐	☐
Am I Proud of my workout for the day?..................	☐	☐
Did I snack Healthy today?......................................	☐	☐

Snacks and Beverages:	Candy, Sugar, or Salt Coated	Dipping Sauce	Healthy or Unhealthy

Wild WORKOUT®

Approach Used

□	□	□
Direct Target	Mix & Match	Circuit

Wild WORKOUT® **Exercise**

Exercise	Reps	Sets

Self Evaluation: (Check one) | A+ | A | B | C | D | F |

Hydration
12 oz Glasses of Water

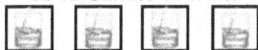

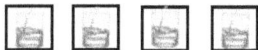

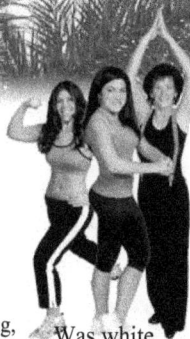

Food	How was it Prepared?	What Dressing, Topping, dipping sauce, or butter was used?	Was white flour or sugar used?

	Yes	No
Did I follow the "Four Secrets of Health" today?.....	☐	☐
Did I keep myself hydrated today?..........................	☐	☐
Am I Proud of my workout for the day?.................	☐	☐
Did I snack Healthy today?..................................	☐	☐

Snacks and Beverages:	Candy, Sugar, or Salt Coated	Dipping Sauce	Healthy or Unhealthy

Wild WORKOUT®

Approach Used

☐ Direct Target   ☐ Mix & Match   ☐ Circuit

Wild WORKOUT® **Exercise**

Exercise	Reps	Sets

Self Evaluation: (Check one) ☐ A+   ☐ A   ☐ B   ☐ C   ☐ D   ☐ F

Hydration
12 oz Glasses of Water

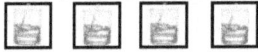

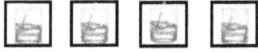

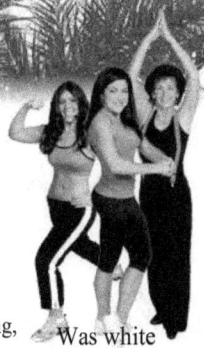

☐	☐	☐	☐
☐	☐	☐	☐

Food	How was it Prepared?	What Dressing, Topping, dipping sauce, or butter was used?	Was white flour or sugar used?

	Yes	No
Did I follow the "Four Secrets of Health" today?.....	☐	☐
Did I keep myself hydrated today?............................	☐	☐
Am I Proud of my workout for the day?..................	☐	☐
Did I snack Healthy today?.....................................	☐	☐

Snacks and Beverages:	Candy, Sugar, or Salt Coated	Dipping Sauce	Healthy or Unhealthy

Wild **WORKOUT**®

Approach Used

☐ Direct Target ☐ Mix & Match ☐ Circuit

Wild **WORKOUT**® **Exercise**

Exercise	Reps	Sets

Self Evaluation: (Check one) ☐ A+ ☐ A ☐ B ☐ C ☐ D ☐ F

Hydration
12 oz Glasses of Water

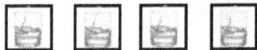

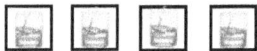

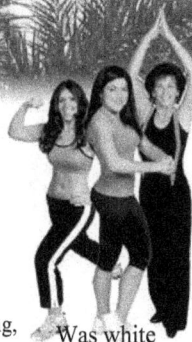

☐ ☐ ☐ ☐

☐ ☐ ☐ ☐

Food	How was it Prepared?	What Dressing, Topping, dipping sauce, or butter was used?	Was white flour or sugar used?

	Yes	No
Did I follow the "Four Secrets of Health" today?.....	☐	☐
Did I keep myself hydrated today?...........................	☐	☐
Am I Proud of my workout for the day?..................	☐	☐
Did I snack Healthy today?....................................	☐	☐

Snacks and Beverages:	Candy, Sugar, or Salt Coated	Dipping Sauce	Healthy or Unhealthy

Wild WORKOUT.

Approach Used

☐	☐	☐
Direct Target	Mix & Match	Circuit

Wild WORKOUT. Exercise

Exercise	Reps	Sets

Self Evaluation: (Check one) [A+] [A] [B] [C] [D] [F]

Hydration
12 oz Glasses of Water

☐ ☐ ☐ ☐

☐ ☐ ☐ ☐

Food	How was it Prepared?	What Dressing, Topping, dipping sauce, or butter was used?	Was white flour or sugar used?

	Yes	No
Did I follow the "Four Secrets of Health" today?.....	☐	☐
Did I keep myself hydrated today?...........................	☐	☐
Am I Proud of my workout for the day?.................	☐	☐
Did I snack Healthy today?......................................	☐	☐

Snacks and Beverages:	Candy, Sugar, or Salt Coated	Dipping Sauce	Healthy or Unhealthy

23

Wild WORKOUT®

Approach Used

☐ ☐ ☐

Direct Target   Mix & Match   Circuit

Wild WORKOUT® **Exercise**

Exercise	Reps	Sets

Self Evaluation: (Check one) ☐ A+ ☐ A ☐ B ☐ C ☐ D ☐ F

1:6

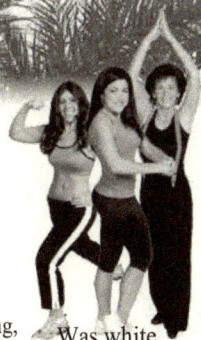

Hydration
12 oz Glasses of Water

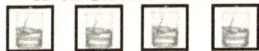

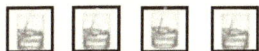

Food	How was it Prepared?	What Dressing, Topping, dipping sauce, or butter was used?	Was white flour or sugar used?

	Yes	No
Did I follow the "Four Secrets of Health" today?.....	☐	☐
Did I keep myself hydrated today?...........................	☐	☐
Am I Proud of my workout for the day?..................	☐	☐
Did I snack Healthy today?......................................	☐	☐

Snacks and Beverages:	Candy, Sugar, or Salt Coated	Dipping Sauce	Healthy or Unhealthy

Wild WORKOUT®

Approach Used

☐ Direct Target ☐ Mix & Match ☐ Circuit

Wild WORKOUT® Exercise

Exercise	Reps	Sets

Self Evaluation: (Check one) ☐ A+ ☐ A ☐ B ☐ C ☐ D ☐ F

Hydration
12 oz Glasses of Water

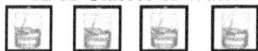

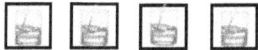

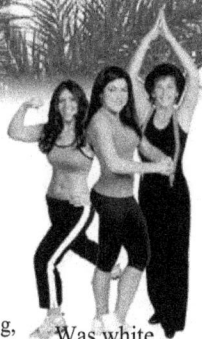

Food	How was it Prepared?	What Dressing, Topping, dipping sauce, or butter was used?	Was white flour or sugar used?

	Yes	No
Did I follow the "Four Secrets of Health" today?.....	☐	☐
Did I keep myself hydrated today?...........................	☐	☐
Am I Proud of my workout for the day?................	☐	☐
Did I snack Healthy today?......................................	☐	☐

Snacks and Beverages:	Candy, Sugar, or Salt Coated	Dipping Sauce	Healthy or Unhealthy

Wild **WORKOUT**®

Approach Used

☐ Direct Target ☐ Mix & Match ☐ Circuit

Wild **WORKOUT**® **Exercise** | **Reps** | **Sets**

Exercise	Reps	Sets

Self Evaluation: (Check one) ☐ A+ ☐ A ☐ B ☐ C ☐ D ☐ F

Hydration
12 oz Glasses of Water

Food	How was it Prepared?	What Dressing, Topping, dipping sauce, or butter was used?	Was white flour or sugar used?

	Yes	No
Did I follow the "Four Secrets of Health" today?.....	☐	☐
Did I keep myself hydrated today?..........................	☐	☐
Am I Proud of my workout for the day?.................	☐	☐
Did I snack Healthy today?....................................	☐	☐

Snacks and Beverages:	Candy, Sugar, or Salt Coated	Dipping Sauce	Healthy or Unhealthy

Wild WORKOUT®

Approach Used ☐ ☐ ☐

Direct Target   Mix & Match   Circuit

Wild WORKOUT® Exercise

Exercise	Reps	Sets

Self Evaluation: (Check one) ☐ A+ ☐ A ☐ B ☐ C ☐ D ☐ F

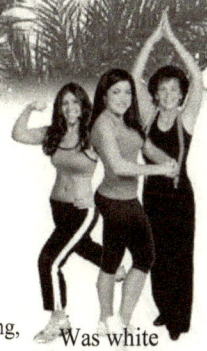

Hydration
12 oz Glasses of Water

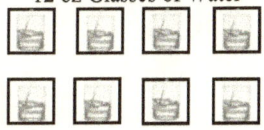

Food	How was it Prepared?	What Dressing, Topping, dipping sauce, or butter was used?	Was white flour or sugar used?

	Yes	No
Did I follow the "Four Secrets of Health" today?.....	☐	☐
Did I keep myself hydrated today?...........................	☐	☐
Am I Proud of my workout for the day?..................	☐	☐
Did I snack Healthy today?.......................................	☐	☐

Snacks and Beverages:	Candy, Sugar, or Salt Coated	Dipping Sauce	Healthy or Unhealthy

Week 2 Day 3

Date: ___ / ___ / ___

Wild **WORKOUT**®

Approach Used

☐	☐	☐
Direct Target	Mix & Match	Circuit

Wild WORKOUT® Exercise	Reps	Sets

Self Evaluation: (Check one) A+ A B C D F

_____

_____

_____

_____

Hydration
12 oz Glasses of Water

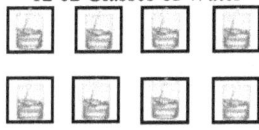

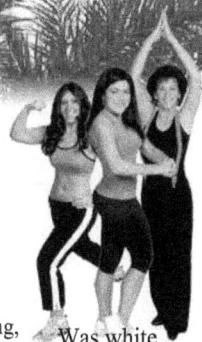

Food	How was it Prepared?	What Dressing, Topping, dipping sauce, or butter was used?	Was white flour or sugar used?

	Yes	No
Did I follow the "Four Secrets of Health" today?.....	☐	☐
Did I keep myself hydrated today?...........................	☐	☐
Am I Proud of my workout for the day?..................	☐	☐
Did I snack Healthy today?......................................	☐	☐

Snacks and Beverages:	Candy, Sugar, or Salt Coated	Dipping Sauce	Healthy or Unhealthy

Wild WORKOUT®

Approach Used

☐ Direct Target ☐ Mix & Match ☐ Circuit

Wild WORKOUT® **Exercise**

Exercise	Reps	Sets

Self Evaluation: (Check one) ☐ A+ ☐ A ☐ B ☐ C ☐ D ☐ F

Hydration
12 oz Glasses of Water

Food	How was it Prepared?	What Dressing, Topping, dipping sauce, or butter was used?	Was white flour or sugar used?

	Yes	No
Did I follow the "Four Secrets of Health" today?.....	☐	☐
Did I keep myself hydrated today?...........................	☐	☐
Am I Proud of my workout for the day?..................	☐	☐
Did I snack Healthy today?.....................................	☐	☐

Snacks and Beverages:	Candy, Sugar, or Salt Coated	Dipping Sauce	Healthy or Unhealthy

Week 2 Day 5

Date: ___ / ___ / ___

Wild WORKOUT®

Approach Used

☐ Direct Target   ☐ Mix & Match   ☐ Circuit

Wild WORKOUT® **Exercise**

Exercise	Reps	Sets

Self Evaluation: (Check one) ☐ A+ ☐ A ☐ B ☐ C ☐ D ☐ F

Hydration
12 oz Glasses of Water

Food	How was it Prepared?	What Dressing, Topping, dipping sauce, or butter was used?	Was white flour or sugar used?

	Yes	No
Did I follow the "Four Secrets of Health" today?.....	☐	☐
Did I keep myself hydrated today?...........................	☐	☐
Am I Proud of my workout for the day?..................	☐	☐
Did I snack Healthy today?.....................................	☐	☐

Snacks and Beverages:	Candy, Sugar, or Salt Coated	Dipping Sauce	Healthy or Unhealthy

Wild WORKOUT®

Approach Used

☐ Direct Target   ☐ Mix & Match   ☐ Circuit

Wild WORKOUT® **Exercise**

Exercise	Reps	Sets

Self Evaluation: (Check one) ☐ A+ ☐ A ☐ B ☐ C ☐ D ☐ F

Hydration
12 oz Glasses of Water

Food	How was it Prepared?	What Dressing, Topping, dipping sauce, or butter was used?	Was white flour or sugar used?

	Yes	No
Did I follow the "Four Secrets of Health" today?.....	☐	☐
Did I keep myself hydrated today?...........................	☐	☐
Am I Proud of my workout for the day?..................	☐	☐
Did I snack Healthy today?.....................................	☐	☐

Snacks and Beverages:	Candy, Sugar, or Salt Coated	Dipping Sauce	Healthy or Unhealthy

Wild WORKOUT®

Approach Used

☐ Direct Target ☐ Mix & Match ☐ Circuit

Wild WORKOUT® **Exercise**

Exercise	Reps	Sets

Self Evaluation: (Check one) A+ A B C D F

Hydration
12 oz Glasses of Water

☐ ☐ ☐ ☐

☐ ☐ ☐ ☐

Food	How was it Prepared?	What Dressing, Topping, dipping sauce, or butter was used?	Was white flour or sugar used?

	Yes	No
Did I follow the "Four Secrets of Health" today?.....	☐	☐
Did I keep myself hydrated today?...........................	☐	☐
Am I Proud of my workout for the day?..................	☐	☐
Did I snack Healthy today?......................................	☐	☐

Snacks and Beverages:	Candy, Sugar, or Salt Coated	Dipping Sauce	Healthy or Unhealthy

Wild WORKOUT®

Approach Used

☐ Direct Target ☐ Mix & Match ☐ Circuit

Wild WORKOUT® **Exercise** | **Reps** | **Sets**

Exercise	Reps	Sets

Self Evaluation: (Check one) ☐ A+ ☐ A ☐ B ☐ C ☐ D ☐ F

Hydration
12 oz Glasses of Water

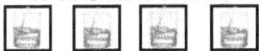

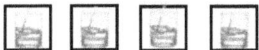

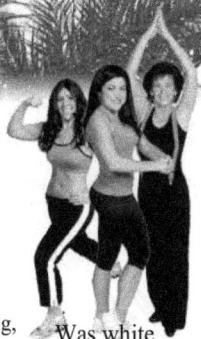

☐ ☐ ☐ ☐

☐ ☐ ☐ ☐

Food	How was it Prepared?	What Dressing, Topping, dipping sauce, or butter was used?	Was white flour or sugar used?

	Yes	No
Did I follow the "Four Secrets of Health" today?.....	☐	☐
Did I keep myself hydrated today?...........................	☐	☐
Am I Proud of my workout for the day?..................	☐	☐
Did I snack Healthy today?.....................................	☐	☐

Snacks and Beverages:	Candy, Sugar, or Salt Coated	Dipping Sauce	Healthy or Unhealthy

43

Wild **WORKOUT**®

Approach Used

Direct Target	Mix & Match	Circuit

Wild **WORKOUT**® **Exercise**

Exercise	Reps	Sets

Self Evaluation: (Check one) A+ A B C D F

_____

_____

_____

_____

_____

Hydration
12 oz Glasses of Water

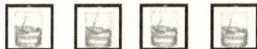

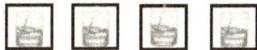

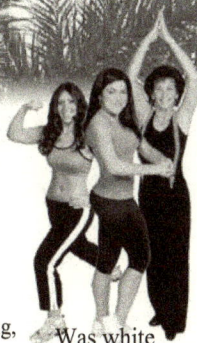

Food	How was it Prepared?	What Dressing, Topping, dipping sauce, or butter was used?	Was white flour or sugar used?

	Yes	No
Did I follow the "Four Secrets of Health" today?.....	☐	☐
Did I keep myself hydrated today?...........................	☐	☐
Am I Proud of my workout for the day?.................	☐	☐
Did I snack Healthy today?.....................................	☐	☐

Snacks and Beverages:	Candy, Sugar, or Salt Coated	Dipping Sauce	Healthy or Unhealthy

Wild WORKOUT ®

Approach Used

☐ Direct Target ☐ Mix & Match ☐ Circuit

Wild WORKOUT ® **Exercise**	Reps	Sets

Self Evaluation: (Check one) ☐ A+ ☐ A ☐ B ☐ C ☐ D ☐ F

Hydration
12 oz Glasses of Water

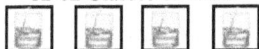

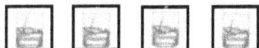

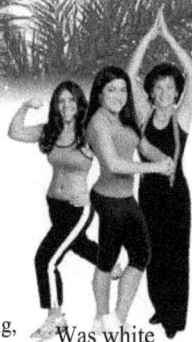

☐ ☐ ☐ ☐

☐ ☐ ☐ ☐

Food	How was it Prepared?	What Dressing, Topping, dipping sauce, or butter was used?	Was white flour or sugar used?

	Yes	No
Did I follow the "Four Secrets of Health" today?.....	☐	☐
Did I keep myself hydrated today?...........................	☐	☐
Am I Proud of my workout for the day?..................	☐	☐
Did I snack Healthy today?......................................	☐	☐

Snacks and Beverages:	Candy, Sugar, or Salt Coated	Dipping Sauce	Healthy or Unhealthy

Wild WORKOUT ®

Approach Used

☐ Direct Target ☐ Mix & Match ☐ Circuit

Wild WORKOUT ® **Exercise**

Exercise	Reps	Sets

Self Evaluation: (Check one) ☐ A+ ☐ A ☐ B ☐ C ☐ D ☐ F

_____
_____
_____
_____
_____

Hydration
12 oz Glasses of Water

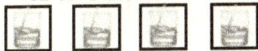

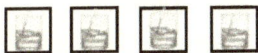

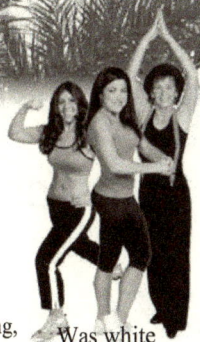

☐ ☐ ☐ ☐

☐ ☐ ☐ ☐

Food	How was it Prepared?	What Dressing, Topping, dipping sauce, or butter was used?	Was white flour or sugar used?

	Yes	No
Did I follow the "Four Secrets of Health" today?.....	☐	☐
Did I keep myself hydrated today?...........................	☐	☐
Am I Proud of my workout for the day?..................	☐	☐
Did I snack Healthy today?.......................................	☐	☐

Snacks and Beverages:	Candy, Sugar, or Salt Coated	Dipping Sauce	Healthy or Unhealthy

Wild WORKOUT®

Approach Used

☐ Direct Target   ☐ Mix & Match   ☐ Circuit

Wild WORKOUT® **Exercise**

Exercise	Reps	Sets

Self Evaluation: (Check one) ☐ A+ ☐ A ☐ B ☐ C ☐ D ☐ F

Hydration
12 oz Glasses of Water

☐ ☐ ☐ ☐

☐ ☐ ☐ ☐

Food	How was it Prepared?	What Dressing, Topping, dipping sauce, or butter was used?	Was white flour or sugar used?

	Yes	No
Did I follow the "Four Secrets of Health" today?.....	☐	☐
Did I keep myself hydrated today?...........................	☐	☐
Am I Proud of my workout for the day?.................	☐	☐
Did I snack Healthy today?.....................................	☐	☐

Snacks and Beverages:	Candy, Sugar, or Salt Coated	Dipping Sauce	Healthy or Unhealthy

51

Wild WORKOUT®

Approach Used

☐ Direct Target ☐ Mix & Match ☐ Circuit

Wild WORKOUT® Exercise

Exercise	Reps	Sets

Self Evaluation: (Check one) ☐ A+ ☐ A ☐ B ☐ C ☐ D ☐ F

Hydration
12 oz Glasses of Water

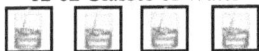

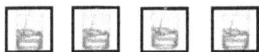

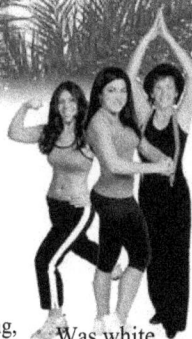

☐ ☐ ☐ ☐

☐ ☐ ☐ ☐

Food	How was it Prepared?	What Dressing, Topping, dipping sauce, or butter was used?	Was white flour or sugar used?

	Yes	No
Did I follow the "Four Secrets of Health" today?.....	☐	☐
Did I keep myself hydrated today?...........................	☐	☐
Am I Proud of my workout for the day?..................	☐	☐
Did I snack Healthy today?.....................................	☐	☐

Snacks and Beverages:	Candy, Sugar, or Salt Coated	Dipping Sauce	Healthy or Unhealthy

Week 3 Day 7

Date: ___ / ___ / ___

Wild WORKOUT ®

Approach Used

☐	☐	☐
Direct Target	Mix & Match	Circuit

Wild WORKOUT ® Exercise

Exercise	Reps	Sets

Self Evaluation: (Check one) ☐ A+ ☐ A ☐ B ☐ C ☐ D ☐ F

3:7

Hydration
12 oz Glasses of Water

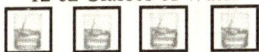

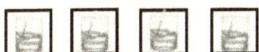

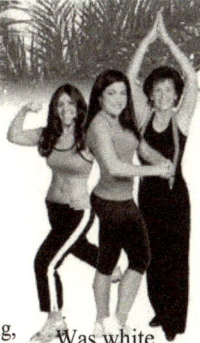

☐ ☐ ☐ ☐

☐ ☐ ☐ ☐

Food	How was it Prepared?	What Dressing, Topping, dipping sauce, or butter was used?	Was white flour or sugar used?

	Yes	No
Did I follow the "Four Secrets of Health" today?.....	☐	☐
Did I keep myself hydrated today?...........................	☐	☐
Am I Proud of my workout for the day?..................	☐	☐
Did I snack Healthy today?.....................................	☐	☐

Snacks and Beverages:	Candy, Sugar, or Salt Coated	Dipping Sauce	Healthy or Unhealthy

Wild WORKOUT®

Approach Used

☐ Direct Target ☐ Mix & Match ☐ Circuit

Wild WORKOUT® **Exercise**

Exercise	Reps	Sets

Self Evaluation: (Check one) ☐ A+ ☐ A ☐ B ☐ C ☐ D ☐ F

_____
_____
_____
_____
_____

Hydration
12 oz Glasses of Water

Food	How was it Prepared?	What Dressing, Topping, dipping sauce, or butter was used?	Was white flour or sugar used?

	Yes	No
Did I follow the "Four Secrets of Health" today?.....	☐	☐
Did I keep myself hydrated today?...........................	☐	☐
Am I Proud of my workout for the day?.................	☐	☐
Did I snack Healthy today?.....................................	☐	☐

Snacks and Beverages:	Candy, Sugar, or Salt Coated	Dipping Sauce	Healthy or Unhealthy

Week 4 Day 2

Date: ___ / ___ / ___

Wild WORKOUT ®

Approach Used

☐ Direct Target ☐ Mix & Match ☐ Circuit

Wild WORKOUT ® Exercise

Exercise	Reps	Sets

Self Evaluation: (Check one) ☐ A+ ☐ A ☐ B ☐ C ☐ D ☐ F

_____
_____
_____
_____
_____

Hydration

12 oz Glasses of Water

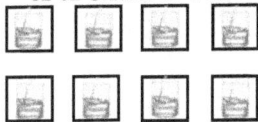

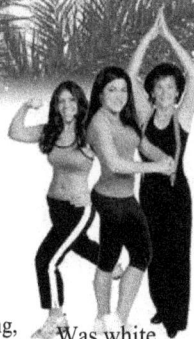

Food	How was it Prepared?	What Dressing, Topping, dipping sauce, or butter was used?	Was white flour or sugar used?

	Yes	No
Did I follow the "Four Secrets of Health" today?.....	☐	☐
Did I keep myself hydrated today?...........................	☐	☐
Am I Proud of my workout for the day?..................	☐	☐
Did I snack Healthy today?.....................................	☐	☐

Snacks and Beverages:	Candy, Sugar, or Salt Coated	Dipping Sauce	Healthy or Unhealthy

Week 4 Day 3

Date: ___ / ___ / ___

Wild WORKOUT ®

Approach Used

☐	☐	☐
Direct Target	Mix & Match	Circuit

Wild WORKOUT ® **Exercise**

Exercise	Reps	Sets

Self Evaluation: (Check one) ☐ A+ ☐ A ☐ B ☐ C ☐ D ☐ F

_____

_____

_____

_____

_____

Hydration
12 oz Glasses of Water

☐ ☐ ☐ ☐

☐ ☐ ☐ ☐

Food	How was it Prepared?	What Dressing, Topping, dipping sauce, or butter was used?	Was white flour or sugar used?

	Yes	No
Did I follow the "Four Secrets of Health" today?.....	☐	☐
Did I keep myself hydrated today?...........................	☐	☐
Am I Proud of my workout for the day?..................	☐	☐
Did I snack Healthy today?......................................	☐	☐

Snacks and Beverages:	Candy, Sugar, or Salt Coated	Dipping Sauce	Healthy or Unhealthy

61

Wild **WORKOUT**®

Approach Used

☐	☐	☐
Direct Target	Mix & Match	Circuit

Wild **WORKOUT**® **Exercise**

Exercise	Reps	Sets

Self Evaluation: (Check one) ☐ A+ ☐ A ☐ B ☐ C ☐ D ☐ F

_____

_____

_____

_____

_____

Hydration
12 oz Glasses of Water

☐ ☐ ☐ ☐

☐ ☐ ☐ ☐

Food	How was it Prepared?	What Dressing, Topping, dipping sauce, or butter was used?	Was white flour or sugar used?

	Yes	No
Did I follow the "Four Secrets of Health" today?	☐	☐
Did I keep myself hydrated today?	☐	☐
Am I Proud of my workout for the day?	☐	☐
Did I snack Healthy today?	☐	☐

Snacks and Beverages:	Candy, Sugar, or Salt Coated	Dipping Sauce	Healthy or Unhealthy

Week 4 Day 5

Date: ___ / ___ / ___

Wild WORKOUT®

Approach Used

☐ Direct Target ☐ Mix & Match ☐ Circuit

Wild WORKOUT® Exercise

Exercise	Reps	Sets

Self Evaluation: (Check one) ☐ A+ ☐ A ☐ B ☐ C ☐ D ☐ F

Hydration
12 oz Glasses of Water

Food	How was it Prepared?	What Dressing, Topping, dipping sauce, or butter was used?	Was white flour or sugar used?

	Yes	No
Did I follow the "Four Secrets of Health" today?.....	☐	☐
Did I keep myself hydrated today?...........................	☐	☐
Am I Proud of my workout for the day?..................	☐	☐
Did I snack Healthy today?......................................	☐	☐

Snacks and Beverages:	Candy, Sugar, or Salt Coated	Dipping Sauce	Healthy or Unhealthy

Week 4 Day 6

Date: ___ / ___ / ___

Wild WORKOUT®

Approach Used

☐ Direct Target ☐ Mix & Match ☐ Circuit

Wild WORKOUT® Exercise	Reps	Sets

Self Evaluation: (Check one) ☐ A+ ☐ A ☐ B ☐ C ☐ D ☐ F

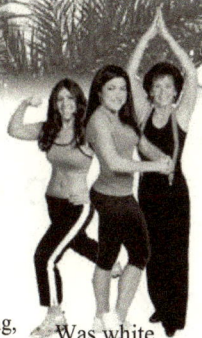

Hydration
12 oz Glasses of Water

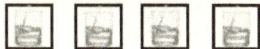

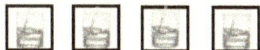

Food	How was it Prepared?	What Dressing, Topping, dipping sauce, or butter was used?	Was white flour or sugar used?

	Yes	No
Did I follow the "Four Secrets of Health" today?.....	☐	☐
Did I keep myself hydrated today?............................	☐	☐
Am I Proud of my workout for the day?..................	☐	☐
Did I snack Healthy today?......................................	☐	☐

Snacks and Beverages:	Candy, Sugar, or Salt Coated	Dipping Sauce	Healthy or Unhealthy

Wild WORKOUT®

Approach Used

☐ Direct Target ☐ Mix & Match ☐ Circuit

Wild WORKOUT® **Exercise**	Reps	Sets

Self Evaluation: (Check one) ☐ A+ ☐ A ☐ B ☐ C ☐ D ☐ F

_____

_____

_____

_____

_____

Hydration
12 oz Glasses of Water

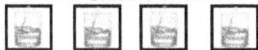

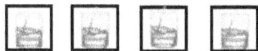

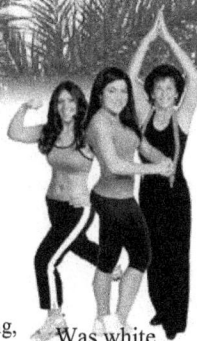

☐ ☐ ☐ ☐

☐ ☐ ☐ ☐

Food	How was it Prepared?	What Dressing, Topping, dipping sauce, or butter was used?	Was white flour or sugar used?

	Yes	No
Did I follow the "Four Secrets of Health" today?.....	☐	☐
Did I keep myself hydrated today?...........................	☐	☐
Am I Proud of my workout for the day?.................	☐	☐
Did I snack Healthy today?.....................................	☐	☐

Snacks and Beverages:	Candy, Sugar, or Salt Coated	Dipping Sauce	Healthy or Unhealthy

Week 5 Day 1

Date: ___ / ___ / ___

Wild **WORKOUT**®

Approach Used

☐ Direct Target ☐ Mix & Match ☐ Circuit

Wild **WORKOUT**® **Exercise**	Reps	Sets

Self Evaluation: (Check one) ☐ A+ ☐ A ☐ B ☐ C ☐ D ☐ F

Hydration
12 oz Glasses of Water

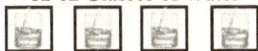

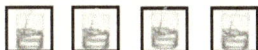

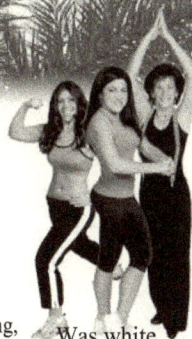

Food	How was it Prepared?	What Dressing, Topping, dipping sauce, or butter was used?	Was white flour or sugar used?

	Yes	No
Did I follow the "Four Secrets of Health" today?.....	☐	☐
Did I keep myself hydrated today?...........................	☐	☐
Am I Proud of my workout for the day?..................	☐	☐
Did I snack Healthy today?......................................	☐	☐

Snacks and Beverages:	Candy, Sugar, or Salt Coated	Dipping Sauce	Healthy or Unhealthy

Week 5 Day 2

Date: ___ / ___ / ___

Wild WORKOUT®

Approach Used

☐ Direct Target   ☐ Mix & Match   ☐ Circuit

Wild WORKOUT® Exercise	Reps	Sets

Self Evaluation: (Check one) ☐ A+ ☐ A ☐ B ☐ C ☐ D ☐ F

_____
_____
_____
_____
_____

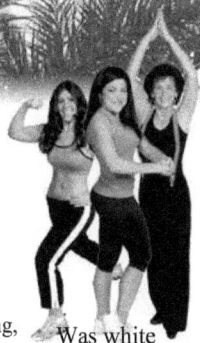

Hydration
12 oz Glasses of Water

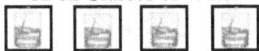

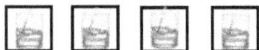

Food	How was it Prepared?	What Dressing, Topping, dipping sauce, or butter was used?	Was white flour or sugar used?

	Yes	No
Did I follow the "Four Secrets of Health" today?	☐	☐
Did I keep myself hydrated today?	☐	☐
Am I Proud of my workout for the day?	☐	☐
Did I snack Healthy today?	☐	☐

Snacks and Beverages:	Candy, Sugar, or Salt Coated	Dipping Sauce	Healthy or Unhealthy

Week 5 Day 3

Date: ___ / ___ / ___

Wild **WORKOUT** ®

Approach Used

☐ Direct Target ☐ Mix & Match ☐ Circuit

Wild **WORKOUT** ® **Exercise**

Exercise	Reps	Sets

Self Evaluation: (Check one) ☐ A+ ☐ A ☐ B ☐ C ☐ D ☐ F

Hydration
12 oz Glasses of Water

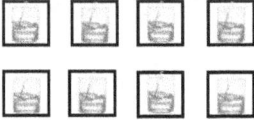

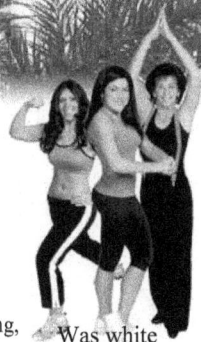

☐ ☐ ☐ ☐

☐ ☐ ☐ ☐

Food	How was it Prepared?	What Dressing, Topping, dipping sauce, or butter was used?	Was white flour or sugar used?

	Yes	No
Did I follow the "Four Secrets of Health" today?.....	☐	☐
Did I keep myself hydrated today?...........................	☐	☐
Am I Proud of my workout for the day?..................	☐	☐
Did I snack Healthy today?......................................	☐	☐

Snacks and Beverages:	Candy, Sugar, or Salt Coated	Dipping Sauce	Healthy or Unhealthy

Week 5 Day 4

Date: ___ / ___ / ___

Wild WORKOUT®

Approach Used

☐ Direct Target ☐ Mix & Match ☐ Circuit

Wild WORKOUT® Exercise

Exercise	Reps	Sets

Self Evaluation: (Check one) ☐ A+ ☐ A ☐ B ☐ C ☐ D ☐ F

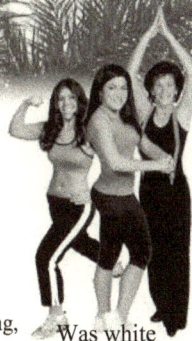

Hydration
12 oz Glasses of Water

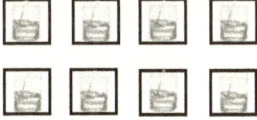

☐ ☐ ☐ ☐

☐ ☐ ☐ ☐

Food	How was it Prepared?	What Dressing, Topping, dipping sauce, or butter was used?	Was white flour or sugar used?

	Yes	No
Did I follow the "Four Secrets of Health" today?.....	☐	☐
Did I keep myself hydrated today?...........................	☐	☐
Am I Proud of my workout for the day?.................	☐	☐
Did I snack Healthy today?......................................	☐	☐

Snacks and Beverages:	Candy, Sugar, or Salt Coated	Dipping Sauce	Healthy or Unhealthy

Week 5 Day 5

Date: ___ / ___ / ___

Wild WORKOUT®

Approach Used

☐ Direct Target ☐ Mix & Match ☐ Circuit

Wild WORKOUT® Exercise

Exercise	Reps	Sets

Self Evaluation: (Check one) ☐ A+ ☐ A ☐ B ☐ C ☐ D ☐ F

Hydration
12 oz Glasses of Water

☐ ☐ ☐ ☐

☐ ☐ ☐ ☐

Food	How was it Prepared?	What Dressing, Topping, dipping sauce, or butter was used?	Was white flour or sugar used?

	Yes	No
Did I follow the "Four Secrets of Health" today?.....	☐	☐
Did I keep myself hydrated today?...........................	☐	☐
Am I Proud of my workout for the day?..................	☐	☐
Did I snack Healthy today?......................................	☐	☐

Snacks and Beverages:	Candy, Sugar, or Salt Coated	Dipping Sauce	Healthy or Unhealthy

Week 5 Day 6

Date: ___ / ___ / ___

Wild WORKOUT®

Approach Used

☐ Direct Target ☐ Mix & Match ☐ Circuit

Wild WORKOUT® Exercise	Reps	Sets

Self Evaluation: (Check one) ☐ A+ ☐ A ☐ B ☐ C ☐ D ☐ F

Hydration
12 oz Glasses of Water

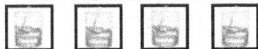

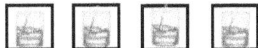

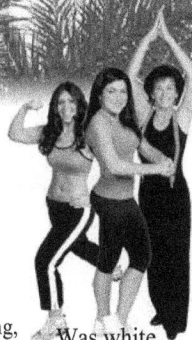

☐ ☐ ☐ ☐

☐ ☐ ☐ ☐

Food	How was it Prepared?	What Dressing, Topping, dipping sauce, or butter was used?	Was white flour or sugar used?

	Yes	No
Did I follow the "Four Secrets of Health" today?.....	☐	☐
Did I keep myself hydrated today?...........................	☐	☐
Am I Proud of my workout for the day?.................	☐	☐
Did I snack Healthy today?......................................	☐	☐

Snacks and Beverages:	Candy, Sugar, or Salt Coated	Dipping Sauce	Healthy or Unhealthy

Wild WORKOUT®

Approach Used

☐ ☐ ☐

Direct   Mix &   Circuit
Target   Match

Wild WORKOUT® **Exercise**

	Reps	Sets

Self Evaluation: (Check one) A+ A B C D F

Hydration
12 oz Glasses of Water

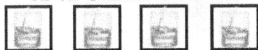

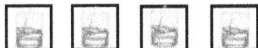

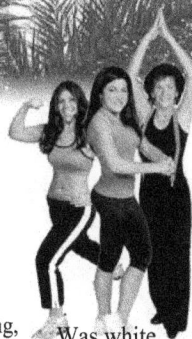

Food	How was it Prepared?	What Dressing, Topping, dipping sauce, or butter was used?	Was white flour or sugar used?

	Yes	No
Did I follow the "Four Secrets of Health" today?.....	☐	☐
Did I keep myself hydrated today?..........................	☐	☐
Am I Proud of my workout for the day?.................	☐	☐
Did I snack Healthy today?.....................................	☐	☐

Snacks and Beverages:	Candy, Sugar, or Salt Coated	Dipping Sauce	Healthy or Unhealthy

Wild WORKOUT®

Approach Used

☐ Direct Target ☐ Mix & Match ☐ Circuit

Wild WORKOUT® **Exercise**

Exercise	Reps	Sets

Self Evaluation: (Check one) ☐ A+ ☐ A ☐ B ☐ C ☐ D ☐ F

Hydration
12 oz Glasses of Water

☐ ☐ ☐ ☐

☐ ☐ ☐ ☐

Food	How was it Prepared?	What Dressing, Topping, dipping sauce, or butter was used?	Was white flour or sugar used?

	Yes	No
Did I follow the "Four Secrets of Health" today?.....	☐	☐
Did I keep myself hydrated today?...........................	☐	☐
Am I Proud of my workout for the day?..................	☐	☐
Did I snack Healthy today?.....................................	☐	☐

Snacks and Beverages:	Candy, Sugar, or Salt Coated	Dipping Sauce	Healthy or Unhealthy

85

Wild WORKOUT®

Approach Used

☐ Direct Target ☐ Mix & Match ☐ Circuit

Wild WORKOUT® Exercise	Reps	Sets

Self Evaluation: (Check one) ☐ A+ ☐ A ☐ B ☐ C ☐ D ☐ F

_____

_____

_____

_____

_____

Hydration
12 oz Glasses of Water

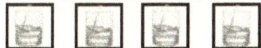

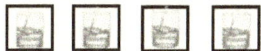

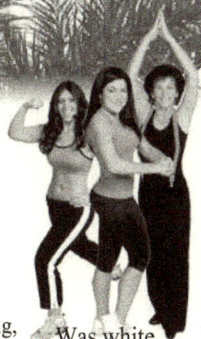

☐ ☐ ☐ ☐

☐ ☐ ☐ ☐

Food	How was it Prepared?	What Dressing, Topping, dipping sauce, or butter was used?	Was white flour or sugar used?

	Yes	No
Did I follow the "Four Secrets of Health" today?.....	☐	☐
Did I keep myself hydrated today?...........................	☐	☐
Am I Proud of my workout for the day?..................	☐	☐
Did I snack Healthy today?......................................	☐	☐

Snacks and Beverages:	Candy, Sugar, or Salt Coated	Dipping Sauce	Healthy or Unhealthy

Wild WORKOUT®

Approach Used

☐ Direct Target ☐ Mix & Match ☐ Circuit

Wild WORKOUT® Exercise | Reps | Sets

Exercise	Reps	Sets

Self Evaluation: (Check one) ☐ A+ ☐ A ☐ B ☐ C ☐ D ☐ F

6:3

Hydration
12 oz Glasses of Water

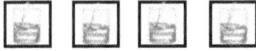

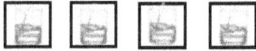

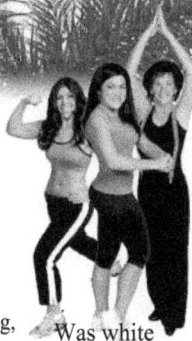

Food	How was it Prepared?	What Dressing, Topping, dipping sauce, or butter was used?	Was white flour or sugar used?

	Yes	No
Did I follow the "Four Secrets of Health" today?.....	☐	☐
Did I keep myself hydrated today?...........................	☐	☐
Am I Proud of my workout for the day?.................	☐	☐
Did I snack Healthy today?......................................	☐	☐

Snacks and Beverages:	Candy, Sugar, or Salt Coated	Dipping Sauce	Healthy or Unhealthy

Wild WORKOUT ®

Approach Used

☐ Direct Target ☐ Mix & Match ☐ Circuit

Wild WORKOUT® **Exercise**	Reps	Sets

Self Evaluation: (Check one) A+ A B C D F

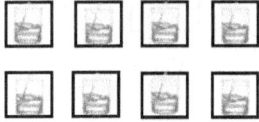

Hydration
12 oz Glasses of Water

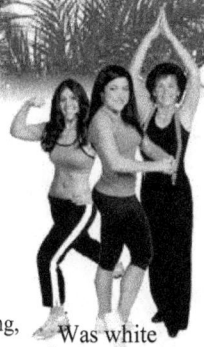

Food	How was it Prepared?	What Dressing, Topping, dipping sauce, or butter was used?	Was white flour or sugar used?

	Yes	No
Did I follow the "Four Secrets of Health" today?.....	☐	☐
Did I keep myself hydrated today?...........................	☐	☐
Am I Proud of my workout for the day?..................	☐	☐
Did I snack Healthy today?......................................	☐	☐

Snacks and Beverages:	Candy, Sugar, or Salt Coated	Dipping Sauce	Healthy or Unhealthy

Wild WORKOUT®

Approach Used

☐ Direct Target   ☐ Mix & Match   ☐ Circuit

Wild WORKOUT® Exercise	Reps	Sets

Self Evaluation: (Check one) ☐ A+ ☐ A ☐ B ☐ C ☐ D ☐ F

Hydration
12 oz Glasses of Water

☐ ☐ ☐ ☐

☐ ☐ ☐ ☐

Food	How was it Prepared?	What Dressing, Topping, dipping sauce, or butter was used?	Was white flour or sugar used?

	Yes	No
Did I follow the "Four Secrets of Health" today?.....	☐	☐
Did I keep myself hydrated today?...........................	☐	☐
Am I Proud of my workout for the day?.................	☐	☐
Did I snack Healthy today?......................................	☐	☐

Snacks and Beverages:	Candy, Sugar, or Salt Coated	Dipping Sauce	Healthy or Unhealthy

Week 6 Day 6

Date: ___ / ___ / ___

Wild **WORKOUT**®

Approach Used

☐ Direct Target   ☐ Mix & Match   ☐ Circuit

Wild **WORKOUT**® **Exercise**	Reps	Sets

Self Evaluation: (Check one) ☐ A+ ☐ A ☐ B ☐ C ☐ D ☐ F

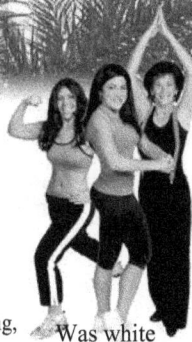

Hydration
12 oz Glasses of Water

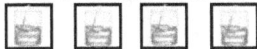

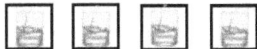

Food	How was it Prepared?	What Dressing, Topping, dipping sauce, or butter was used?	Was white flour or sugar used?

	Yes	No
Did I follow the "Four Secrets of Health" today?.....	☐	☐
Did I keep myself hydrated today?..........................	☐	☐
Am I Proud of my workout for the day?.................	☐	☐
Did I snack Healthy today?......................................	☐	☐

Snacks and Beverages:	Candy, Sugar, or Salt Coated	Dipping Sauce	Healthy or Unhealthy

95

Wild WORKOUT.

Approach Used

☐	☐	☐
Direct Target	Mix & Match	Circuit

Wild WORKOUT. **Exercise**

Exercise	Reps	Sets

Self Evaluation: (Check one) A+ | A | B | C | D | F

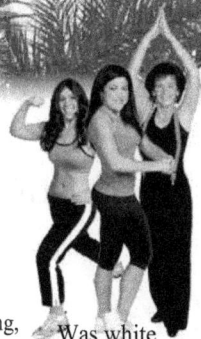

Hydration
12 oz Glasses of Water

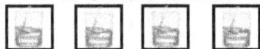

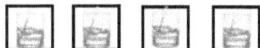

Food	How was it Prepared?	What Dressing, Topping, dipping sauce, or butter was used?	Was white flour or sugar used?

	Yes	No
Did I follow the "Four Secrets of Health" today?.....	☐	☐
Did I keep myself hydrated today?..........................	☐	☐
Am I Proud of my workout for the day?..................	☐	☐
Did I snack Healthy today?.....................................	☐	☐

Snacks and Beverages:	Candy, Sugar, or Salt Coated	Dipping Sauce	Healthy or Unhealthy

Wild WORKOUT®

Approach Used

☐ Direct Target ☐ Mix & Match ☐ Circuit

Wild WORKOUT® **Exercise**

Exercise	Reps	Sets

Self Evaluation: (Check one) ☐ A+ ☐ A ☐ B ☐ C ☐ D ☐ F

_____

_____

_____

_____

7:1

Hydration
12 oz Glasses of Water

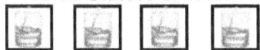

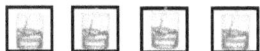

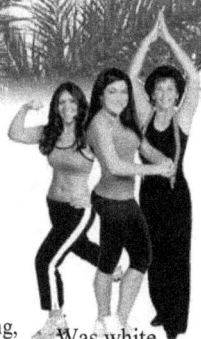

☐ ☐ ☐ ☐

☐ ☐ ☐ ☐

Food	How was it Prepared?	What Dressing, Topping, dipping sauce, or butter was used?	Was white flour or sugar used?

	Yes	No
Did I follow the "Four Secrets of Health" today?.....	☐	☐
Did I keep myself hydrated today?............................	☐	☐
Am I Proud of my workout for the day?.................	☐	☐
Did I snack Healthy today?......................................	☐	☐

Snacks and Beverages:	Candy, Sugar, or Salt Coated	Dipping Sauce	Healthy or Unhealthy

Week 7 Day 2

Date: ___ / ___ / ___

Wild WORKOUT®

Approach Used

Direct Target	Mix & Match	Circuit

Wild WORKOUT® **Exercise**

Exercise	Reps	Sets

Self Evaluation: (Check one) A+ | A | B | C | D | F

Hydration
12 oz Glasses of Water

Food	How was it Prepared?	What Dressing, Topping, dipping sauce, or butter was used?	Was white flour or sugar used?

	Yes	No
Did I follow the "Four Secrets of Health" today?.....	☐	☐
Did I keep myself hydrated today?............................	☐	☐
Am I Proud of my workout for the day?.................	☐	☐
Did I snack Healthy today?.....................................	☐	☐

Snacks and Beverages:	Candy, Sugar, or Salt Coated	Dipping Sauce	Healthy or Unhealthy

Wild WORKOUT®

Approach Used

☐ Direct Target ☐ Mix & Match ☐ Circuit

Wild WORKOUT® **Exercise**

Exercise	Reps	Sets

Self Evaluation: (Check one)

☐ A+ ☐ A ☐ B ☐ C ☐ D ☐ F

7:3

Hydration
12 oz Glasses of Water

Food	How was it Prepared?	What Dressing, Topping, dipping sauce, or butter was used?	Was white flour or sugar used?

	Yes	No
Did I follow the "Four Secrets of Health" today?.....	☐	☐
Did I keep myself hydrated today?.......................	☐	☐
Am I Proud of my workout for the day?..................	☐	☐
Did I snack Healthy today?..............................	☐	☐

Snacks and Beverages:	Candy, Sugar, or Salt Coated	Dipping Sauce	Healthy or Unhealthy

Wild WORKOUT®

Approach Used

☐	☐	☐
Direct Target	Mix & Match	Circuit

Wild WORKOUT® Exercise

Exercise	Reps	Sets

Self Evaluation: (Check one) [A+] [A] [B] [C] [D] [F]

Hydration
12 oz Glasses of Water

Food	How was it Prepared?	What Dressing, Topping, dipping sauce, or butter was used?	Was white flour or sugar used?

	Yes	No
Did I follow the "Four Secrets of Health" today?.....	☐	☐
Did I keep myself hydrated today?...........................	☐	☐
Am I Proud of my workout for the day?.................	☐	☐
Did I snack Healthy today?.....................................	☐	☐

Snacks and Beverages:	Candy, Sugar, or Salt Coated	Dipping Sauce	Healthy or Unhealthy

Wild WORKOUT®

Approach Used

☐ Direct Target ☐ Mix & Match ☐ Circuit

Wild WORKOUT® **Exercise**	Reps	Sets

Self Evaluation: (Check one) A+ A B C D F

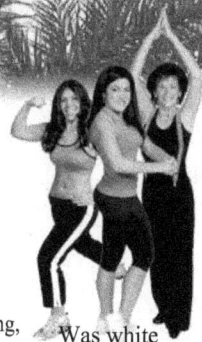

Hydration
12 oz Glasses of Water

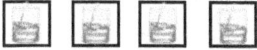

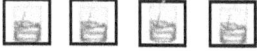

Food	How was it Prepared?	What Dressing, Topping, dipping sauce, or butter was used?	Was white flour or sugar used?

	Yes	No
Did I follow the "Four Secrets of Health" today?.....	☐	☐
Did I keep myself hydrated today?...........................	☐	☐
Am I Proud of my workout for the day?..................	☐	☐
Did I snack Healthy today?......................................	☐	☐

Snacks and Beverages:	Candy, Sugar, or Salt Coated	Dipping Sauce	Healthy or Unhealthy

Wild WORKOUT®

Approach Used

☐ Direct Target ☐ Mix & Match ☐ Circuit

Wild WORKOUT® Exercise

Exercise	Reps	Sets

Self Evaluation: (Check one) ☐ A+ ☐ A ☐ B ☐ C ☐ D ☐ F

Hydration
12 oz Glasses of Water

Food	How was it Prepared?	What Dressing, Topping, dipping sauce, or butter was used?	Was white flour or sugar used?

	Yes	No
Did I follow the "Four Secrets of Health" today?.....	☐	☐
Did I keep myself hydrated today?...........................	☐	☐
Am I Proud of my workout for the day?.................	☐	☐
Did I snack Healthy today?......................................	☐	☐

Snacks and Beverages:	Candy, Sugar, or Salt Coated	Dipping Sauce	Healthy or Unhealthy

109

Wild WORKOUT®

Approach Used

☐ Direct Target ☐ Mix & Match ☐ Circuit

Wild WORKOUT® **Exercise**

Exercise	Reps	Sets

Self Evaluation: (Check one) ☐ A+ ☐ A ☐ B ☐ C ☐ D ☐ F

_____

_____

_____

_____

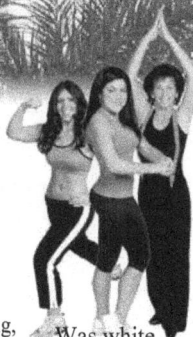

Hydration
12 oz Glasses of Water

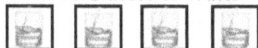

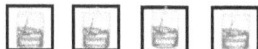

Food	How was it Prepared?	What Dressing, Topping, dipping sauce, or butter was used?	Was white flour or sugar used?

	Yes	No
Did I follow the "Four Secrets of Health" today?.....	☐	☐
Did I keep myself hydrated today?...........................	☐	☐
Am I Proud of my workout for the day?.................	☐	☐
Did I snack Healthy today?.....................................	☐	☐

Snacks and Beverages:	Candy, Sugar, or Salt Coated	Dipping Sauce	Healthy or Unhealthy

Week 8 Day 1

Date: ___ / ___ / ___

Wild WORKOUT®

Approach Used ☐ ☐ ☐

Direct Target   Mix & Match   Circuit

Wild WORKOUT® Exercise

Exercise	Reps	Sets

Self Evaluation: (Check one) ☐ A+ ☐ A ☐ B ☐ C ☐ D ☐ F

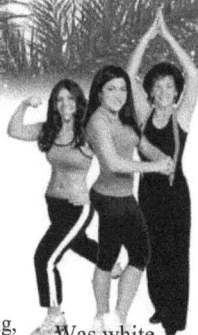

Hydration
12 oz Glasses of Water

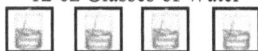 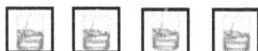

Food	How was it Prepared?	What Dressing, Topping, dipping sauce, or butter was used?	Was white flour or sugar used?

	Yes	No
Did I follow the "Four Secrets of Health" today?.....	☐	☐
Did I keep myself hydrated today?...........................	☐	☐
Am I Proud of my workout for the day?..................	☐	☐
Did I snack Healthy today?...................................	☐	☐

Snacks and Beverages:	Candy, Sugar, or Salt Coated	Dipping Sauce	Healthy or Unhealthy

Wild WORKOUT.

Approach Used

Direct Target	Mix & Match	Circuit

Wild WORKOUT. Exercise

Exercise	Reps	Sets

Self Evaluation: (Check one) A+ A B C D F

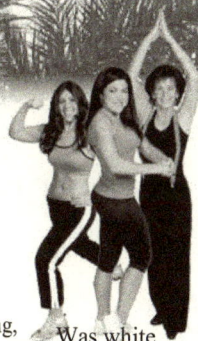

Hydration
12 oz Glasses of Water

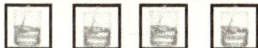

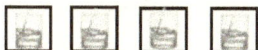

Food	How was it Prepared?	What Dressing, Topping, dipping sauce, or butter was used?	Was white flour or sugar used?

	Yes	No
Did I follow the "Four Secrets of Health" today?.....	☐	☐
Did I keep myself hydrated today?............................	☐	☐
Am I Proud of my workout for the day?..................	☐	☐
Did I snack Healthy today?......................................	☐	☐

Snacks and Beverages:	Candy, Sugar, or Salt Coated	Dipping Sauce	Healthy or Unhealthy

115

Wild WORKOUT®

Approach Used

☐ ☐ ☐

Direct   Mix &   Circuit
Target   Match

Wild WORKOUT® **Exercise** | **Reps** | **Sets**

	Reps	Sets

Self Evaluation: (Check one) A+ A B C D F

_____

WORKOUT BEAUTYFLEX

Hydration
12 oz Glasses of Water

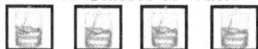

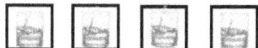

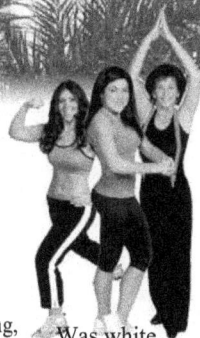

Food	How was it Prepared?	What Dressing, Topping, dipping sauce, or butter was used?	Was white flour or sugar used?

	Yes	No
Did I follow the "Four Secrets of Health" today?.....	☐	☐
Did I keep myself hydrated today?............................	☐	☐
Am I Proud of my workout for the day?..................	☐	☐
Did I snack Healthy today?.....................................	☐	☐

Snacks and Beverages:	Candy, Sugar, or Salt Coated	Dipping Sauce	Healthy or Unhealthy

Wild **WORKOUT**®

Approach Used

☐ Direct Target ☐ Mix & Match ☐ Circuit

Wild **WORKOUT**® **Exercise**	Reps	Sets

Self Evaluation: (Check one) ☐ A+ ☐ A ☐ B ☐ C ☐ D ☐ F

Hydration
12 oz Glasses of Water

Food	How was it Prepared?	What Dressing, Topping, dipping sauce, or butter was used?	Was white flour or sugar used?

	Yes	No
Did I follow the "Four Secrets of Health" today?.....	☐	☐
Did I keep myself hydrated today?............................	☐	☐
Am I Proud of my workout for the day?..................	☐	☐
Did I snack Healthy today?......................................	☐	☐

Snacks and Beverages:	Candy, Sugar, or Salt Coated	Dipping Sauce	Healthy or Unhealthy

Week 8 Day 5

Date: ___ / ___ / ___

Wild WORKOUT®

Approach Used

☐ Direct Target ☐ Mix & Match ☐ Circuit

Wild WORKOUT® **Exercise** | **Reps** | **Sets**

Exercise	Reps	Sets

Self Evaluation: (Check one) ☐ A+ ☐ A ☐ B ☐ C ☐ D ☐ F

Hydration
12 oz Glasses of Water

Food	How was it Prepared?	What Dressing, Topping, dipping sauce, or butter was used?	Was white flour or sugar used?

	Yes	No
Did I follow the "Four Secrets of Health" today?.....	☐	☐
Did I keep myself hydrated today?...........................	☐	☐
Am I Proud of my workout for the day?..................	☐	☐
Did I snack Healthy today?.....................................	☐	☐

Snacks and Beverages:	Candy, Sugar, or Salt Coated	Dipping Sauce	Healthy or Unhealthy

Wild **WORKOUT**®

Approach Used

☐ Direct Target ☐ Mix & Match ☐ Circuit

Wild **WORKOUT**® **Exercise**

Exercise	Reps	Sets

Self Evaluation: (Check one) ☐ A+ ☐ A ☐ B ☐ C ☐ D ☐ F

Hydration
12 oz Glasses of Water

Food	How was it Prepared?	What Dressing, Topping, dipping sauce, or butter was used?	Was white flour or sugar used?

	Yes	No
Did I follow the "Four Secrets of Health" today?.....	☐	☐
Did I keep myself hydrated today?...........................	☐	☐
Am I Proud of my workout for the day?.................	☐	☐
Did I snack Healthy today?....................................	☐	☐

Snacks and Beverages:	Candy, Sugar, or Salt Coated	Dipping Sauce	Healthy or Unhealthy

123

Wild WORKOUT®

Approach Used

☐	☐	☐
Direct Target	Mix & Match	Circuit

Wild WORKOUT® **Exercise**

Exercise	Reps	Sets

Self Evaluation: (Check one) A+ ☐ A ☐ B ☐ C ☐ D ☐ F ☐

Hydration
12 oz Glasses of Water

☐ ☐ ☐ ☐

☐ ☐ ☐ ☐

Food	How was it Prepared?	What Dressing, Topping, dipping sauce, or butter was used?	Was white flour or sugar used?

	Yes	No
Did I follow the "Four Secrets of Health" today?.....	☐	☐
Did I keep myself hydrated today?...........................	☐	☐
Am I Proud of my workout for the day?..................	☐	☐
Did I snack Healthy today?.....................................	☐	☐

Snacks and Beverages:	Candy, Sugar, or Salt Coated	Dipping Sauce	Healthy or Unhealthy